The Art Of Dark Feminine Seduction

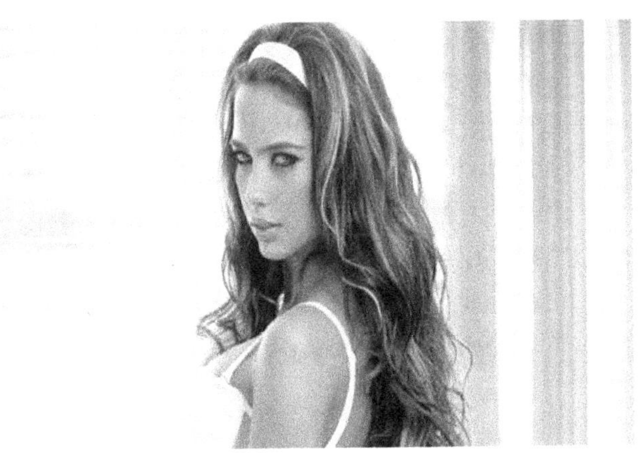

Embrace Your Feminine Power, Navigate the Male Psyche, and Cultivate Irresistible Magnetism.

Natasha Nice

Table of Contents

INTRODUCTION

In the shadows of society's expectations and norms lies a realm shrouded in mystery and allure—the realm of the Dark Feminine. It's a place where power and passion intertwine, where secrets are whispered in the dead of night and desires are unleashed with abandon. In this introduction, we embark on a journey to unveil the enigmatic allure of the Dark Feminine—a journey that promises to awaken the senses and ignite the soul.

As we step into the darkness, we shed the confines of societal conditioning and embrace the raw, unbridled essence of our feminine nature. It's a journey of self-discovery and empowerment, where we confront the shadows within ourselves and emerge stronger, more vibrant, and more alive than ever before. With each step, we peel back the layers of illusion to reveal the truth that lies at our core: we are powerful, we are passionate, and we are unstoppable.

But the Dark Feminine is more than just a force to be reckoned with—it's a source of wisdom, guidance, and transformation. It's the fierce protectress who guards our deepest desires and the gentle nurturer who cradles our dreams in her embrace. It's the embodiment of our darkest fears and our greatest aspirations, all woven together in a tapestry of strength and vulnerability.

In unveiling the Dark Feminine, we embrace the full spectrum of our humanity—the light and the shadow, the beauty and the beast. We recognize that true power lies not in suppressing our darker impulses, but in embracing them with open arms and integrating them into the fabric of our being. It's a journey of self-acceptance and self-love, where we learn to honor every aspect of ourselves without judgment or shame.

So join me, dear reader, as we journey into the depths of the unknown and embrace the wild, untamed beauty of the Dark Feminine. Together, we will discover the power that lies within us all and unleash it upon the world with fearless abandon. For in the darkness, we find not only our greatest fears, but also our greatest strength.

Chapter 1: Embracing Your Feminine Power

In the quiet moments of reflection, amidst the chaos of everyday life, there exists a gentle whisper—a reminder of the innate strength that resides within each and every woman. It's a strength born of resilience, nurtured by adversity, and tempered by the fires of experience. In this journey of self-discovery, we begin by acknowledging the power that lies dormant within us, waiting to be unleashed upon the world.

As we peel back the layers of doubt and uncertainty, we uncover the raw, unbridled essence of our feminine power. It's a power that defies definition, transcending the boundaries of time and space to touch the hearts and minds of all who encounter it. It's the quiet confidence that radiates from within, the unwavering belief in ourselves and our abilities, and the unshakable resolve to overcome any obstacle that stands in our way.

But embracing our feminine power is more than just acknowledging our strength—it's about embracing our vulnerability as well. It's about recognizing that true power lies not in the absence of fear, but in the courage to face it head-on and emerge victorious. It's about honoring the parts of ourselves that we often deem unworthy or weak, and finding strength in our imperfections.

Within each woman beats the heart of a goddess—an ethereal being of light and beauty, whose radiance illuminates the darkest corners of the universe. It's a beauty that transcends physical appearance, radiating from within and captivating all who are fortunate enough to bask in its glow. In embracing our unique feminine energy, we embrace the essence of who we are: powerful, sensual, and utterly irresistible.

Our feminine energy is a force to be reckoned with—a magnetic pull that draws others to us with an irresistible allure. It's the gentle sway of our hips as we move through the world, the softness of our touch that leaves a trail of sparks in its wake, and the intoxicating scent of our presence that lingers long after we're gone. It's a power that is uniquely ours, waiting to be harnessed and unleashed upon the world with wild abandon.

Deep within the recesses of our souls lies a secret waiting to be discovered—a hidden wellspring of magic and enchantment that lies dormant until called upon. It's the essence of our inner enchantress, a seductive siren whose allure knows no bounds. In unleashing our inner enchantress, we tap into the depths of our desires and unleash them upon the world with reckless abandon.

Our inner enchantress is a force of nature—a tempest of passion and desire that sweeps through the hearts and minds of all who dare to cross her path. She is wild and untamed, a creature of instinct and intuition who knows no boundaries or limitations. In embracing her, we embrace the fullness of our feminine power and embrace the intoxicating thrill of being alive.

But unleashing our inner enchantress requires courage and vulnerability. It requires us to let go of our inhibitions and embrace the fullness of who we are without reservation. It's about owning our desires and embracing our passions with open arms, unapologetically and without shame. It's a journey of self-discovery and self-expression, where we learn to honor our deepest desires and embrace our truest selves with wild abandon.

Recognizing Your Strength Within

In the quiet moments of reflection, amidst the ebb and flow of daily life, there is a whisper—a gentle reminder of the reservoir of strength that resides within each woman. It is a strength forged in the crucible of experience, shaped by trials and tribulations, and tempered by the fires of adversity.

As we embark on the journey of recognizing our strength within, we peel back the layers of doubt and insecurity to reveal the core of our being—a wellspring of resilience and fortitude that defies expectation. It is the quiet voice within us that refuses to be silenced, the indomitable spirit that rises from the ashes of defeat, and the unwavering belief in our own capabilities.

But recognizing our strength within is not merely about acknowledging our past triumphs or overcoming obstacles—it is about embracing the inherent power that lies dormant within us, waiting to be unleashed upon the world. It is about recognizing that true strength is not measured by the absence of fear or doubt, but by the courage to confront our deepest fears and insecurities head-on.

In recognizing our strength within, we also come to understand the importance of self-compassion and self-care. It is about acknowledging our own worth and value, and treating ourselves with the kindness and respect that we deserve. It is about embracing our flaws and imperfections, and understanding that they are an integral part of what makes us uniquely beautiful and resilient.

So let us embrace the strength that lies within us, dear reader, and let it guide us on our journey of self-discovery and empowerment. For it is in recognizing and harnessing our own inner power that we truly become unstoppable.

Embracing Your Unique Feminine Energy

Within every woman lies a spectrum of energy as diverse and rich as the colors of the earth. It's a dynamic force, flowing through us, shaping our essence, and painting the world with our presence.

Embracing our unique feminine energy is like stepping into the depths of our soul, where every facet of our being shines with its own brilliance. It's a journey of self-discovery, peeling away layers of conditioning to reveal the raw, untamed beauty within. It's about honoring every aspect of ourselves—the softness and strength, the vulnerability and resilience—without holding back.

At its core, embracing our feminine energy is about surrender and empowerment. It's about letting go of control and allowing ourselves to flow with life's natural rhythms. It's trusting our intuition, embracing our sensuality, and celebrating the sacredness of our sexuality without inhibition.

But it also requires courage—the courage to explore our creativity, embrace our wildness, and trust in our instincts. It's about reclaiming our bodies as vessels of divine expression and honoring the wisdom that resides within us.

So let's embrace our unique feminine energy with open hearts and open minds. Let's revel in the beauty of our diversity and shine brightly in the world, illuminating every corner with the radiant essence of our femininity.

Unleashing Your Inner Enchantress

Deep within the caverns of our soul, there exists a dormant power—a primal force of seduction and allure waiting to be awakened. It is the essence of our inner enchantress, a mysterious muse whose whispers stir the very fabric of reality.

To unleash our inner enchantress is to delve into the depths of our desires, to embrace the forbidden fruits of our imagination, and to surrender to the wild, untamed passions that course through our veins.

It is a journey of self-discovery and self-mastery, where we confront our deepest fears and insecurities, and emerge stronger, more confident, and more radiant than ever before.

But it is also a journey fraught with danger and temptation, for to unleash our inner enchantress is to dance on the razor's edge between light and darkness, ecstasy and agony, creation and destruction.

Yet, it is in this delicate balance that we find our true power—the power to shape our own destiny, to command the forces of the universe, and to manifest our wildest dreams with a mere flick of our wrist.

So let us embrace the darkness and the light, the chaos and the order, the beauty and the beast within us, and let us unleash our inner enchantress with fierce determination and unwavering grace. For in doing so, we reclaim our birthright as divine goddesses, creators of our own reality, and rulers of our own destiny.

The Dance of Desire: Unleashing Your Inner Enchantress

In the sultry embrace of the night, we find ourselves drawn into a dance—a dance of desire, of seduction, of ecstasy. It is the dance of our inner enchantress, weaving her spell of enchantment with every sway of her hips, every flick of her wrist, every whispered promise of pleasure.

To unleash our inner enchantress is to surrender to the primal urges that lie dormant within us—to embrace the intoxicating allure of our own sensuality, and to revel in the ecstasy of our own divine femininity.

It is a journey of self-discovery and self-expression, where we shed the shackles of societal expectation and embrace the fullness of who we are. It is a journey of liberation, of empowerment, of transformation.

But it is also a journey of vulnerability and courage, for to unleash our inner enchantress is to confront the shadows that lurk within us—to face our deepest fears and insecurities, and to embrace them with open arms.

Yet, it is in this vulnerability that we find our greatest strength—the strength to embrace our desires without shame or inhibition, to express ourselves authentically and unapologetically, and to claim our rightful place as sovereign goddesses of our own destiny.

So let us embrace the dance of desire, dear sisters, and let us unleash our inner enchantress with wild abandon and unwavering confidence. For in doing so, we reclaim our power, our passion, and our purpose, and emerge from the shadows reborn—a radiant goddess, fierce and free.

Seduction as Art: Unleashing Your Inner Enchantress

Seduction is not merely a game—it is an art form, a dance of desire that transcends the boundaries of time and space. It is the art of unleashing our inner enchantress, of weaving spells of enchantment with every glance, every touch, every whispered word.

To master the art of seduction is to tap into the primal forces of creation—to harness the power of our own feminine energy and channel it with precision and grace. It is a journey of self-discovery and self-expression, where we explore the depths of our desires and embrace the fullness of who we are.

But it is also a journey of courage and vulnerability, for to seduce is to expose ourselves to the gaze of others—to lay bare our deepest longings and desires, and to risk rejection and heartache in the process.

Yet, it is in this vulnerability that we find our greatest strength—the strength to embrace our desires without shame or inhibition, to express ourselves authentically and unapologetically, and to claim our rightful place as sovereign goddesses of our own destiny.

So let us embrace the art of seduction, dear sisters, and let us unleash our inner enchantress with wild abandon and unwavering confidence. For in doing so, we reclaim our power, our passion, and our purpose, and emerge from the shadows reborn—a radiant goddess, fierce and free.

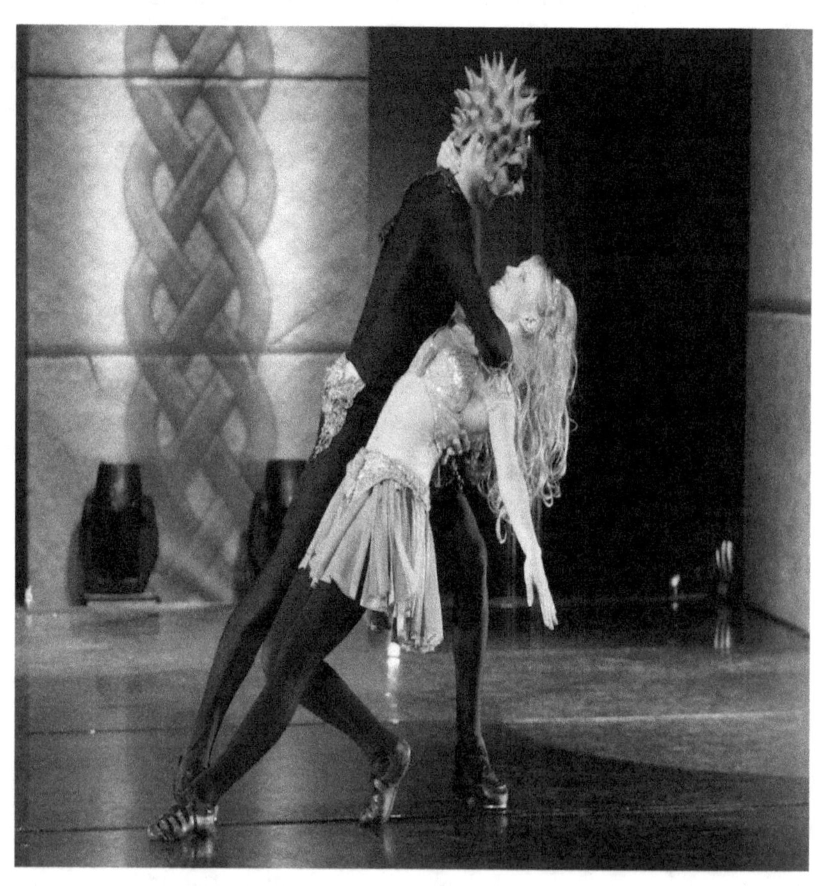

16

Chapter 2: Navigating the Male Psyche: Unraveling the Mysteries

Within the labyrinth of the male psyche lies a world of complexity, a tapestry woven with threads of desire, emotion, and instinct. To navigate this intricate landscape is to embark on a journey of discovery—one filled with twists and turns, challenges and triumphs, and a profound understanding of the masculine soul.

As women, we often find ourselves drawn to the enigma of the male psyche, seeking to unravel its mysteries and unlock its secrets. Yet, it is a journey fraught with uncertainty, for the male mind is a labyrinth of contradictions—a delicate balance of strength and vulnerability, confidence and insecurity, passion and fear.

To navigate the male psyche is to navigate a maze of emotions—a landscape shaped by upbringing, culture, and personal experience. It is to understand the nuances of masculine communication, to decipher the language of gestures, tones, and expressions that speak volumes without a word.

But it is also a journey of empathy and compassion, for to truly understand the male psyche is to recognize the depth of its pain, the breadth of its joy, and the complexity of its desires. It is to embrace the vulnerability that lies at its core, to offer support and encouragement in times of need, and to celebrate its victories with genuine admiration and respect.

Yet, navigating the male psyche is not without its challenges, for men are often taught to suppress their emotions, to hide their vulnerabilities, and to mask their true selves behind a facade of strength. It is a journey of breaking down barriers, of peeling back layers of conditioning, and of allowing the authentic self to emerge from the shadows.

But in doing so, we open ourselves to a world of profound connection and intimacy—a world where hearts are laid bare, souls are laid bare, and love flows freely between two kindred spirits. It is a journey of deepening trust, of mutual understanding, and of forging a bond that transcends the limitations of the physical realm.

So let us embark on this journey together, dear sisters, with open hearts and open minds. Let us navigate the male psyche with courage and compassion, with empathy and understanding, and with a profound respect for the mysteries that lie within. For in doing so, we not only unlock the secrets of the masculine soul but also discover the true depths of our own.

Decoding Male Psychology: Understanding the Depths

Within the vast expanse of human psychology, the male mind stands as a landscape of profound complexity—a realm shaped by an array of factors, from biology and upbringing to cultural norms and personal experiences. To decode male psychology is to embark on a journey of exploration and revelation—a journey that delves into the hidden depths of the masculine psyche.

At its core, decoding male psychology demands a thorough examination of the intricate interplay between thoughts, emotions, and behaviors that define the male experience. It necessitates a deep understanding of the societal pressures and expectations that shape masculine identity, as well as the individual nuances that color each man's perception of himself and the world around him.

But beyond the surface lies a world of emotion—a realm often obscured by societal norms and gender stereotypes. Decoding male psychology requires a keen insight into the subtle cues and signals that men use to express themselves, from the nuances of body language to the nuances of verbal communication.

Yet, it is also a journey of introspection and self-discovery, as we confront our own biases and assumptions about masculinity and strive to cultivate a more empathetic and understanding perspective. It is a journey that challenges us to look beyond the surface and embrace the complexity of the human experience, to see beyond the stereotypes and appreciate the unique qualities that make each man who he is.

Ultimately, decoding male psychology is a journey of growth and transformation—a journey that empowers us to build stronger, more authentic relationships, and to forge deeper connections with the men in our lives. It is a journey that invites us to explore the depths of human emotion and vulnerability, and to celebrate the rich tapestry of diversity that defines the human experience.

So let us embark on this journey together, dear sisters, with open hearts and open minds. Let us decode male psychology with curiosity and compassion, with humility and respect, and with a steadfast commitment to understanding the depths of the human soul. In doing so, we not only enrich our own lives but also contribute to a more inclusive, empathetic, and compassionate world.

Understanding Masculine Desires and Needs: Exploring the Depths

In the realm of human relationships, understanding masculine desires and needs is a journey into the heart of masculinity itself—a journey that delves into the depths of male psychology, emotion, and behavior. It is a quest to unravel the intricate layers of masculine identity, to decode the subtle cues and signals that men use to express themselves, and to forge deeper connections based on empathy, understanding, and respect.

At its core, understanding masculine desires and needs requires a willingness to listen, to empathize, and to see beyond the surface. It demands a recognition of the unique challenges and pressures that men face in today's world, from societal expectations and gender stereotypes to personal insecurities and fears. It is a journey of introspection and self-discovery, as we confront our own biases and assumptions about masculinity and strive to cultivate a more empathetic and understanding perspective.

But it is also a journey of exploration and revelation, as we uncover the hidden depths of the male psyche and come to appreciate the rich tapestry of desires and needs that define masculine identity. It is a journey that celebrates the diversity of masculine expression, from the bold and assertive to the gentle and vulnerable, and recognizes that there is no one-size-fits-all approach to understanding male desire.

Ultimately, understanding masculine desires and needs is a journey of growth and transformation—a journey that empowers us to build stronger, more authentic relationships, and to forge deeper connections with the men in our lives. It is a journey that invites us to explore the depths of human emotion and vulnerability, and to celebrate the beauty of human connection in all its forms.

So let us embark on this journey together, dear sisters, with open hearts and open minds. Let us seek to understand masculine desires and needs with curiosity and compassion, with humility and respect, and with a steadfast commitment to building a more inclusive, empathetic, and compassionate world. For in doing so, we not only enrich our own lives but also contribute to a deeper understanding and appreciation of the human experience

The Moonlit Dance: Unveiling Dark Seduction for Authentic Connection

Seduction, in its truest form, isn't about manipulation or fleeting desire. It's an art, a moonlit dance where vulnerability and power intertwine. The Dark Feminine, often misunderstood as manipulative, embodies a potent truth: genuine connection arises from embracing the depths of ourselves.

Shedding the Layers: Embracing Your Shadow

The Dark Feminine isn't sugar-coated sweetness. It's the unapologetic acceptance of your desires, your intuition, and even your anger. It's confronting your shadow self, the hidden aspects you might try to repress. By acknowledging these depths, you become more whole, more magnetic.

The Power of Mystery: Unveiling in Layers

Forget spilling your life story on the first date. The Dark Feminine thrives on intrigue. Let your confidence be a slow burn, an enigma that draws someone in. Share glimpses of your passions, your sensuality, your intellect, but leave room for discovery. This dance of unveiling creates a yearning to know you deeper.

Intuition as Your Guide: Trusting Your Inner Voice

The Dark Feminine honors her intuition. Learn to discern genuine connections from fleeting infatuation. Feel the subtle shifts in energy. Don't be afraid to walk away from situations that don't resonate with your soul. This unwavering trust in your inner compass fosters authenticity and empowers you to attract those who truly align with you.

The Enchantment of Vulnerability: Strength in Softness

The Dark Feminine isn't afraid to be vulnerable. Share your dreams, your anxieties, your deepest desires. This creates a space for genuine connection, a vulnerability that invites your partner to do the same. Strength isn't about coldness; it's about embracing all facets of yourself.

The Art of Self-Love: A Foundation for Healthy Connection

The Dark Feminine knows her worth. You can't give authentic love if you don't love yourself fiercely. Invest in your passions, your growth, your well-being. This self-assured radiance is incredibly attractive, and it sets the foundation for a relationship built on mutual respect and admiration.

Remember: The Dark Feminine isn't about mind games. It's about self-discovery, owning your power, and attracting someone who appreciates the multifaceted you. It's about creating an authentic connection, a dance of vulnerability and strength, bathed in the light of the moon.

Chapter 3:. Cultivating Irresistible Magnetism: Embracing Your Radiance

Within the depths of every woman lies a potent energy—a magnetic force that radiates from her core, drawing others to her with an irresistible allure. Cultivating irresistible magnetism is not merely about external appearance, but about tapping into the innate power that resides within and allowing it to shine forth with unabashed confidence.

At its essence, cultivating irresistible magnetism is a journey of self-discovery and self-love. It is about embracing our unique qualities, quirks, and imperfections, and celebrating them as the very essence of our beauty. It is about cultivating a deep sense of self-assurance and authenticity that transcends societal standards of beauty and radiates from within.

To cultivate irresistible magnetism is to harness the power of our thoughts and beliefs, recognizing that our mindset shapes our reality. It is about cultivating a positive outlook on life, fostering a sense of abundance and gratitude, and exuding an aura of confidence and self-assuredness that is undeniably attractive.

But cultivating irresistible magnetism goes beyond mere confidence—it is about embracing our femininity in all its forms. It is about tapping into our sensuality, our passion, and our innate feminine grace, and allowing them to flow freely through every aspect of our being. It is about embracing our authenticity and vulnerability, and allowing ourselves to be seen and heard in all our raw, unfiltered beauty.

It is also about cultivating a magnetic presence that extends beyond ourselves and touches the lives of those around us. It is about fostering deep connections with others through empathy, compassion, and understanding, and creating a ripple effect of positivity and love wherever we go.

Ultimately, cultivating irresistible magnetism is a journey of empowerment—a journey that allows us to reclaim our power, embrace our radiance, and shine brightly in the world. It is a journey that invites us to step into our full potential, to embrace our uniqueness, and to inspire others to do the same.

So let us embrace this journey with open hearts and open minds, dear sisters, and let us cultivate our irresistible magnetism with grace, confidence, and authenticity. For in doing so, we not only elevate ourselves but also uplift those around us and create a world filled with beauty, love, and boundless possibility.

Enhancing Your Aura of Mystery and Allure

In a world saturated with instant gratification and oversharing, cultivating an aura of mystery and allure can be a powerful tool. It's not about playing games; it's about understanding the magnetic pull of the unseen, the unspoken. It's about creating an invitation for deeper connection, a captivating dance between intrigue and revelation.

The Art of Selective Self-Disclosure:

The Dark Feminine, often associated with enigmatic allure, sheds light on this concept. It's not about hiding who you are; it's about revealing yourself strategically. Share glimpses of your passions, your intellect, your sensuality, like brushstrokes painting a captivating portrait. Leave room for the imagination to dance, for questions to arise, for the desire to know you more fully to take root. Let your confidence be a slow burn, a whisper that promises untold stories.

Confidence: The Foundation of Allure

Confidence isn't about arrogance; it's about embracing your unique essence and worth. Cultivate a quiet self-assuredness that shines through in your body language, your voice, and your gaze. This inner strength fosters an air of self-possession, making you intrinsically interesting and desirable. Invest in yourself – your passions, your skills, your well-being. This self-love radiates outward, creating a magnetism that draws people in.

The Power of Curiosity:

Become an observer, a student of the world and the people around you. Ask thoughtful questions, listen intently, and genuinely seek to understand those you interact with. This piques their interest in return, fostering a sense of connection and intrigue. They'll find themselves wanting to share their stories with you, eager to unveil themselves to the captivating listener you are.

Embrace the Power of Pause:

In an age of instant replies and overcommunication, the power of the pause is often forgotten. Don't feel pressured to respond immediately to messages or invitations. Let anticipation build. This creates a sense of intrigue and allows the other person to invest more emotionally in the connection.

The Allure of the Unpredictable:

While reliability is important, a touch of the unexpected can be incredibly alluring. Don't be afraid to break from routine occasionally. Surprise with a thoughtful gesture, a sudden burst of laughter, or a hidden talent revealed. This unpredictability keeps the other person engaged, eager to see what fascinating layer you might unveil next.

Cultivating an Air of Mystery is not Deception

Remember, the key is authenticity. Don't fabricate stories or create a persona that isn't true to yourself. The allure lies in the genuine you, the layers waiting to be discovered. Embrace your complexities, your passions, your shadows. It's in this rich tapestry that true connection and lasting allure reside.

By mastering the art of selective self-disclosure, cultivating confidence, and embracing a touch of the unpredictable, you can cultivate an aura of mystery and allure that draws people in and fosters genuine connections. Remember, the most captivating stories are the ones that leave the reader yearning for more, and you, my friend, are the author of your own captivating narrative.

Mastering the Art of Seductive Communication: Crafting Your Irresistible Charm

In the intricate dance of human interaction, communication is the key that unlocks the doors to desire, passion, and connection. Mastering the art of seductive communication is not merely about words—it is about crafting an irresistible charm that captivates the mind, stirs the soul, and leaves others spellbound in your presence.

At its essence, mastering the art of seductive communication is a journey of self-awareness and self-expression. It is about understanding the power of your words, your tone, your body language, and your presence, and using them to weave a tapestry of intrigue and fascination that draws others to you with an irresistible pull.

To master the art of seductive communication is to cultivate a deep understanding of human psychology—the subtle nuances of desire, the hidden meanings behind words, and the unspoken language of attraction. It is about tapping into the desires and fantasies that lie dormant within us all, and using them to create a connection that transcends the ordinary.

But mastering the art of seductive communication is also about authenticity and vulnerability. It is about speaking from the heart, sharing your desires and fears openly and honestly, and allowing yourself to be seen and heard in all your raw, unfiltered beauty.

To master the art of seductive communication is to embrace the power of your voice—both literal and metaphorical. It is about speaking with confidence and conviction, using your words to paint a vivid picture of the world you desire, and inviting others to join you on the journey.

But perhaps most importantly, mastering the art of seductive communication is about embracing your own unique charm and charisma. It is about tapping into the wellspring of your inner goddess or god, allowing your authentic self to shine through, and exuding a magnetic presence that draws others to you like moths to a flame.

So let us embark on this journey together, dear friends, with open hearts and open minds. Let us master the art of seductive communication with grace and confidence, trusting in the power of our words and the magic of our presence to captivate and enchant those around us. For in doing so, we not only elevate our own experiences but also create a world filled with passion, connection, and boundless possibility.

Commanding the Room: Mastering the Art of Confidence and Charisma

Confidence and charisma aren't inborn traits; they're skills that can be honed and cultivated. They are the invisible threads that weave together a captivating presence, allowing you to project power, inspire trust, and magnetically draw people in. Here's your roadmap to becoming proficient in this skill:

The Power of Positive Body Language:
The signals your body sends convey a wealth of information even before you speak.Stand tall with open shoulders, a relaxed yet steady gaze, and a hint of a smile. Steer clear of fidgeting or crossing your arms, as these behaviors may indicate feelings of insecurity. Use confident gestures that complement your points, but avoid nervous ticks that distract from your message.

Speak with Conviction:
Project your voice clearly and with a steady tempo. Avoid monotone delivery or nervous upspeak. Vary your vocal inflections to emphasize key points and keep your audience engaged. Enthusiasm is contagious, so let your passion for the topic shine through in your voice.

Become a Master Storyteller:
People connect with stories. Weave anecdotes and relatable examples into your conversations and presentations. This not only makes your message more memorable, but it also allows you to showcase your personality and connect with your audience on a deeper level.

Active Listening: The Art of True Connection
Confidence isn't about dominating the conversation; it's about fostering genuine interaction. Listen intently to what others are saying, make eye contact, and ask thoughtful questions. This demonstrates your respect and

interest, making you a more captivating and trustworthy presence.

Embrace Your Imperfections:
Nobody's perfect, and trying to appear flawless can come across as inauthentic. Acknowledge your mistakes with grace and humor. This self-awareness projects confidence and fosters a sense of connection with your audience, who can relate to your human vulnerabilities.

Dress for the Role You Want:
First impressions matter. Dress in a way that makes you feel confident and powerful, whether it's a sharp suit or a stylish outfit that reflects your personal brand. When you feel good about how you look, it shows in your posture, your demeanor, and your overall charisma.

Cultivate Knowledge and Passion:
Confidence stems from competence. Be well-informed about your field or the topic at hand. Demonstrate your passion and expertise by sharing interesting facts, insights, and experiences. This intellectual depth makes you a captivating conversationalist and a person others seek out for knowledge and inspiration.

Practice Makes Perfect:
Don't wait for a grand opportunity to project confidence. Start small. Practice clear communication and strong body language in

everyday interactions. Volunteer for presentations or take on leadership roles in group projects. The more comfortable you become in various settings, the more naturally confidence and charisma will exude from you.

Remember, confidence and charisma are journeys, not destinations. By embracing these tips and consistently honing your skills, you'll transform yourself into a captivating presence who commands attention and inspires others. You'll become the leader you were meant to be, one powerful interaction at a time.

In the intricate dance of human interaction, communication is the key that unlocks the doors to desire, passion, and connection. Mastering the art of seductive communication is not merely about words—it is about crafting an irresistible charm that captivates the mind, stirs the soul, and leaves others spellbound in your presence.

At its essence, mastering the art of seductive communication is a journey of self-awareness and self-expression. It is about understanding the power of your words, your tone, your body language, and your presence, and using them to weave a tapestry of intrigue and fascination that draws others to you with an irresistible pull.

To master the art of seductive communication is to cultivate a deep understanding of human psychology—the subtle nuances of desire, the hidden meanings behind words, and the unspoken language of attraction. It is about tapping into the desires and fantasies that lie dormant within us all, and using them to create a connection that transcends the ordinary.

But mastering the art of seductive communication is also about authenticity and vulnerability. It is about speaking from the heart, sharing your desires and fears openly and honestly, and allowing yourself to be seen and heard in all your raw, unfiltered beauty.

To master the art of seductive communication is to embrace the power of your voice—both literal and metaphorical. It is about speaking with confidence and conviction, using your words to paint a vivid picture of the world you desire, and inviting others to join you on the journey.

But perhaps most importantly, mastering the art of seductive communication is about embracing your own unique charm and charisma. It is about tapping into the wellspring of your inner goddess or god, allowing your authentic self to shine through, and exuding a magnetic presence that draws others to you like moths to a flame.

Chapter 4: Embracing Self-Reflection and Self-Compassion: Nurturing the Soul

In the quiet corners of our hearts, amidst the chaos of daily life, lies a sacred sanctuary—a space where we can retreat to reflect, to heal, and to reconnect with our true selves. Embracing self-reflection and self-compassion is not merely an act of introspection, but a profound journey of self-discovery and self-love—a journey that invites us to delve deep into the recesses of our soul, to confront our fears and insecurities, and to embrace our vulnerabilities with open arms.

At its core, embracing self-reflection is about cultivating a gentle curiosity—a willingness to explore the depths of our inner landscape, to unravel the layers of conditioning and programming that shape our beliefs and behaviors, and to shine the light of awareness on the shadows that lurk within.

It is about asking ourselves the tough questions, without judgment or condemnation, and being brave enough to sit with the discomfort that arises as we confront our truths. It is about peeling back the layers of our masks and defenses, and allowing ourselves to be seen and heard in all our raw, unfiltered authenticity.

But self-reflection is not merely about looking inward—it is also about looking outward, and recognizing the interconnectedness of all beings. It is about cultivating empathy and compassion for ourselves and others, recognizing that we are all on this journey of life together, navigating the twists and turns of existence with courage and grace.

To embrace self-compassion is to offer ourselves the same kindness and understanding that we would offer to a dear friend. It is about recognizing our inherent worthiness, regardless of our perceived flaws or shortcomings, and extending ourselves the same forgiveness and grace that we would offer to others.

It is about nurturing the wounded parts of ourselves with tenderness and care, and holding space for our pain and suffering with love and compassion. It is about recognizing that we are all human, all imperfect, and all deserving of love and acceptance just as we are.

But perhaps most importantly, embracing self-reflection and self-compassion is about reclaiming our power—the power to heal, to grow, and to transform our lives in ways we never thought possible. It is about recognizing that our greatest strength lies not in perfection, but in our ability to embrace our imperfections with courage and grace, and to emerge from the depths of our struggles with newfound wisdom and resilience.

So let us embark on this journey of self-discovery and self-love, dear friends, with open hearts and open minds. Let us embrace self-reflection and self-compassion with courage and grace, trusting in the wisdom of our hearts and the resilience of our spirits to guide us on this sacred path of healing and transformation. For in doing so, we not only honor ourselves and our own journey, but we also create a ripple effect of love and compassion that touches the lives of all beings, illuminating the path to healing and wholeness for all.

Exploring Your Inner Depths: Plummeting into the Abyss of Self

Beneath the facade we present to the world lies a labyrinthine maze of emotions, memories, and desires—a universe unto itself waiting to be discovered. To embark on the journey of exploring your inner depths is to dare to dive headfirst into the abyss of self, to unravel the tangled threads of your psyche, and to confront the raw, unfiltered truth that lies at the core of your being.

At its essence, exploring your inner depths is a descent into darkness—a courageous exploration of the shadowy recesses of your soul where fears lurk, wounds fester, and secrets hide. It is a journey fraught with peril, for in the depths of the self lie both the demons that torment us and the treasures that sustain us.

It is about peeling back the layers of protection we have erected around our hearts and allowing ourselves to be vulnerable, to feel deeply, and to embrace the full spectrum of human emotion. It is about confronting our deepest fears and insecurities, and finding the courage to face them head-on, knowing that it is only by shining the light of awareness on our shadows that we can truly begin to heal and grow.

To explore your inner depths is to embark on a quest for self-knowledge—a relentless pursuit of truth, meaning, and purpose in a world that often seems chaotic and uncertain. It is about seeking answers to the questions that haunt us, and finding solace in the silence of our own inner knowing.

But exploring your inner depths is not merely about introspection—it is also about connection. It is about recognizing the interconnectedness of all things, and finding unity in the diversity of human experience. It is about forging deep and meaningful connections with others, and recognizing that we are all on this journey of self-discovery together.

It is about tapping into the wellspring of creativity and inspiration that lies within us, and allowing ourselves to be guided by the wisdom of our intuition. It is about embracing the power of imagination and intuition, and trusting in the guidance of our inner voice as we navigate the twists and turns of the inner landscape.

But perhaps most importantly, exploring your inner depths is about embracing the journey itself—the exhilarating highs and the devastating lows, the moments of clarity and the periods of confusion. It is about surrendering to the ebb and flow of life, and allowing ourselves to be swept away by the currents of our own inner truth.

So let us embark on this journey of exploration and self-discovery, dear friends, with open hearts and open minds. Let us embrace the darkness as well as the light, the fear as well as the courage, knowing that it is only by diving deep into the abyss of self that we can truly discover the boundless depths of our own inner wisdom and truth.

Healing Past Wounds and Limiting Beliefs: Liberating the Soul from the Shackles of the Past

Within the labyrinth of our psyche lies a landscape scarred by the echoes of past traumas and the weight of limiting beliefs—a terrain where shadows loom large and wounds fester unseen. To undertake the journey of healing past wounds and limiting beliefs is to embark on a sacred pilgrimage of self-discovery, resilience, and profound transformation—a journey that calls upon us to navigate the depths of our own inner terrain with courage, compassion, and unwavering determination.

At its core, healing past wounds and limiting beliefs is an act of radical self-love—an audacious declaration of our inherent worthiness, deservingness, and capacity for profound healing and growth. It is a courageous excavation of the layers of conditioning, trauma, and societal expectations that have obscured the truth of our essence—the truth that we are whole, worthy, and infinitely deserving of love and belonging.

It is about peeling back the layers of protective armor that we have constructed around our hearts—the shields of denial, avoidance, and numbing that have shielded us from the pain of our past—and allowing ourselves to be vulnerable, raw, and unapologetically human. It is about leaning into the discomfort of our emotions, acknowledging the wounds that lie beneath, and summoning the courage to face them with compassion, tenderness, and radical acceptance.

To heal past wounds and limiting beliefs is to embark on a sacred alchemical process—a mystical journey of transmutation, integration, and rebirth. It is about alchemizing our pain into wisdom, our fear into courage, and our shame into self-compassion. It is about reclaiming the fragmented pieces of ourselves—the parts that we have disowned, rejected, or abandoned—and weaving them back into the tapestry of our being with reverence, grace, and profound love.

It is about challenging the false narratives and outdated scripts that have dictated our lives—the stories of unworthiness, inadequacy, and not-enoughness that have kept us small, stuck, and playing small. It is about rewriting the narrative of our lives from a place of empowerment, sovereignty, and radical self-ownership, and stepping into the fullest expression of our authentic truth with unshakeable confidence, clarity, and purpose.

But perhaps most importantly, healing past wounds and limiting beliefs is about reclaiming our power—the power to liberate ourselves from the shackles of the past, the power to redefine our reality, and the power to co-create a life of joy, purpose, and fulfillment on our own terms. It is about recognizing that our wounds are not our identity, our pain is not our destiny, and our past does not dictate our future.

So let us undertake this journey of healing and self-discovery with open hearts and open minds—with a fierce commitment to our own liberation, transformation, and soulful evolution. Let us embrace the challenges, the breakthroughs, and the sacred mysteries that await us as we traverse the landscapes of our own inner terrain, knowing that it is only by journeying through the darkness that we can emerge into the radiant light of our own true essence.

Embracing Self-Love and Empowerment: The Journey to Unshakable Inner Strength

In the intricate fabric of our existence, there exists a thread of profound significance—an essence that speaks to the very core of our being. It is the essence of self-love and empowerment, woven into the very fabric of our souls, waiting to be unraveled and embraced with unyielding reverence and devotion. To embark on the journey of embracing self-love and empowerment is to embark on a sacred odyssey—a quest that transcends the boundaries of time and space, leading us to the depths of our own hearts and the heights of our own potential.

At its essence, embracing self-love and empowerment is an act of radical defiance—an audacious declaration of our inherent worthiness and our right to stand firmly in our own truth. It is a courageous journey of self-discovery and self-acceptance, inviting us to peel back the layers of conditioning and limitation that have obscured the brilliance of our true essence, and to bask in the radiant light of our own divine presence.

It is about reclaiming our power—the power to define ourselves on our own terms, to honor the whispers of our own hearts, and to walk boldly in the direction of our dreams. It is about recognizing that our worthiness is not contingent upon external validation or approval, but is an intrinsic aspect of our very being—a sacred birthright that can never be diminished or revoked.

To embrace self-love and empowerment is to cultivate a deep and abiding sense of compassion and kindness towards ourselves—a gentle, nurturing embrace that soothes our weary souls, heals our deepest wounds, and reminds us of our inherent perfection and beauty. It is about treating ourselves with the same tenderness, care, and respect that we would offer to a cherished friend or loved one, and honoring our own needs, desires, and aspirations with unwavering devotion and commitment.

But perhaps most importantly, embracing self-love and empowerment is about recognizing that our greatest strength lies not in our ability to control or manipulate external circumstances, but in our capacity to cultivate an unshakeable inner resilience—a resilience that allows us to navigate the ever-changing tides of life with courage, grace, and unwavering resolve.

It is about harnessing the power of our thoughts, beliefs, and intentions to shape our reality, and stepping boldly into the fullness of our authentic truth with unyielding confidence and clarity. It is about standing tall in our own power, speaking our truth with unwavering conviction, and shining our light brightly into the world, knowing that we are worthy, deserving, and capable of creating the life of our dreams.

Self-love and empowerment aren't fleeting feelings; they're the fertile ground from which a fulfilling life flourishes. They are the unshakeable belief in your worth, the unwavering trust in your abilities, and the fierce commitment to your well-being.
Here's your guide to nurturing this transformative inner garden:

The Seed of Self-Compassion:
Self-love begins with self-compassion. We all make mistakes, experience setbacks, and have moments of doubt. Replace harsh self-criticism with nurturing kindness and understanding. Forgive yourself as you would a dear friend. This gentle approach fosters emotional resilience and empowers you to move forward with grace.

Nurturing Positive Self-Talk:
We are constantly bombarded with external messages. However, the most important voice is the one within. Challenge negative self-talk with affirmations that celebrate your strengths and accomplishments. Speak to yourself with the same encouragement and respect you would offer someone you love.

Prioritizing Self-Care:
Self-care isn't selfish; it's essential. Identify activities that replenish your mind, body, and spirit. Whether it's a quiet meditation session, a rejuvenating bath, or a creative pursuit, prioritize these activities. A well-nourished soul is an empowered soul, ready to take on the world.

Setting Healthy Boundaries:
Boundaries are not walls; they're healthy filters. Learn to say "no" to protect your time, energy, and emotional well-being. Don't be afraid to walk away from situations or people that drain you. Setting

boundaries empowers you to prioritize what truly matters and fosters healthier relationships.

Celebrating Your Strengths and Achievements:
Take pride in your accomplishments, big or small. Acknowledge your unique talents and skills. Keep a gratitude journal to document the positive aspects of your life and celebrate your ongoing growth. This self-appreciation fuels your inner fire and empowers you to strive for more.

Embracing Your Whole Self:
Each of us possesses both brightness and darkness within. Instead of trying to suppress your flaws, embrace your complexities. Accepting all aspects of yourself fosters authenticity and inner peace. This self-acceptance empowers you to be true to yourself, attracting genuine connections and opportunities.

Investing in Personal Growth:
Never stop learning and evolving. Read inspiring books, take courses that pique your interest, and step outside your comfort zone. This continuous learning journey keeps your mind sharp, your spirit curious, and empowers you to navigate life's challenges with confidence.
So let us embark on this journey of self-love and empowerment with open hearts and open minds—with a fierce determination to honor the whispers of our own hearts and unleash the fullness of our potential.

Chapter 5: Mastering the Dance of Seduction: Unveiling the Art of Irresistible Charm

In the grand theater of human connection, there exists a delicate dance—a choreography of desire, intrigue, and allure. To embark on the journey of mastering the dance of seduction is to step onto a stage illuminated by the flickering flames of passion and possibility—a stage where every glance, every touch, and every word holds the potential to captivate the hearts and minds of those who dare to participate.

At its essence, mastering the dance of seduction is an art—a subtle alchemy of confidence, charisma, and authenticity that transcends the limitations of language and logic. It is a journey of self-discovery and self-expression, inviting us to explore the depths of our own desires, fears, and vulnerabilities, and to embrace the fullness of our own unique essence with unbridled passion and conviction.

It is about recognizing that seduction is not merely about manipulation or conquest, but about the playful exchange of energy and intention—a dance of mutual attraction and intrigue that unfolds with grace and finesse. It is about understanding the power of presence, the allure of mystery, and the magnetism of authenticity, and using these qualities to create an irresistible aura of charm and allure that draws others to us like moths to a flame.

To master the dance of seduction is to cultivate a deep and intimate connection with ourselves—a connection that allows us to tap into the wellspring of our own desires, passions, and fantasies, and to express them with confidence and clarity. It is about embracing the fullness of our own sensual nature, and allowing ourselves to revel in the pleasures of the senses without shame or inhibition.

But perhaps most importantly, mastering the dance of seduction is about recognizing that true seduction begins within—that the most irresistible charm emanates from a place of self-assuredness, self-respect, and self-love. It is about cultivating a deep and abiding sense of confidence in ourselves and our own worthiness, and allowing this confidence to shine through in every interaction, every gesture, and every word.

It is about understanding that seduction is not about conforming to a certain ideal of beauty or attractiveness, but about embracing the unique beauty and attractiveness that resides within each of us. It is about celebrating our individuality, our authenticity, and our inherent sexiness, and allowing these qualities to shine through in everything we do.

So let us embark on this journey of mastering the dance of seduction with open hearts and open minds—with a fierce determination to embrace our own unique essence and express it with passion and conviction. Let us explore the depths of our desires, the mysteries of our fantasies, and the limitless potential that lies within us, knowing that it is only by mastering the dance of seduction within ourselves that we can truly captivate the hearts and minds of those around us, and create a life filled with passion, pleasure, and boundless possibility.

Crafting Tension and Intrigue: The Subtle Art of Seduction Mastery

In the intricate tapestry of human connection, there exists a subtle dance—a dance of tension and release, of anticipation and desire. To embark on the journey of mastering the dance of seduction is to embrace the art of crafting tension and intrigue—a delicate interplay of subtlety and suggestion that ignites the flames of passion and leaves hearts aflame with longing.

At its essence, creating tension and intrigue is an art form—a symphony of subtle gestures, lingering glances, and tantalizing whispers that stirs the soul and sets the stage for the seductive embrace of desire. It is about understanding the power of anticipation, the allure of the unknown, and the magnetic pull of the forbidden, and using these elements to weave a web of irresistible charm that draws others into our orbit like moths to a flame.

It is about recognizing that seduction is not about overt manipulation or coercion, but about the artful dance of suggestion and suggestion—a dance that invites participation and engagement, rather than resistance or rejection. It is about creating an atmosphere of mystery and excitement, where every interaction is charged with the electric energy of possibility, and every moment is pregnant with the promise of ecstasy.

To craft tension and intrigue is to cultivate a deep and intuitive understanding of the desires and fantasies that lie hidden beneath the surface of our consciousness—to tap into the wellspring of our own passions and vulnerabilities, and to express them with confidence and finesse. It is about embracing the power of anticipation, and allowing ourselves to savor the delicious tension that arises as we teeter on the edge of surrender, knowing that the adventure is equally thrilling as reaching the final destination.

But perhaps most profoundly, crafting tension and intrigue is about recognizing that true seduction is a dance of reciprocity—a mutual exchange of energy and intention that flows effortlessly between partners, creating a dynamic interplay of attraction and desire. It is about listening to the whispers of our own hearts and responding with authenticity and integrity, allowing the seductive energy to unfold organically and authentically.

So let us embark on this journey of crafting tension and intrigue with open hearts and open minds—with a fierce determination to embrace the mystery and magic of the seductive dance, and to surrender to the intoxicating allure of desire. Let us explore the depths of our own passions, the mysteries of our own fantasies, and the boundless potential that lies within us, knowing that it is only by mastering the art of tension and intrigue that we can truly captivate the hearts and minds of those around us, and create a life filled with passion, pleasure, and boundless possibility., now look at this content generate by you, it is not genuine enough and I am not impressed, give me more points on it and do not write in their format or way

Crafting tension and intrigue in the realm of seduction is a multifaceted endeavor that encompasses various elements to entice and captivate both the reader and the potential partner.

Here's a comprehensive exploration of the different facets that contribute to the art of crafting tension and intrigue:

1. Understanding Psychology: Delve into the psychology of desire and anticipation, exploring how humans are wired to respond to mystery and ambiguity. Discuss the role of neurotransmitters like dopamine and adrenaline in heightening arousal and creating a sense of excitement.

2. The Power of Mystery: Dive deep into the allure of mystery and ambiguity, highlighting how leaving certain aspects unknown can fuel curiosity and desire. Discuss strategies for creating intrigue, such as withholding information, using evocative language, or subtly hinting at hidden depths.

3. Sensory Stimulation: Explore the importance of engaging the senses to create a visceral experience that heightens arousal. Discuss techniques for incorporating sensory elements into seductive encounters, from the subtle scent of perfume to the soft touch of silk against the skin, and the tantalizing taste of forbidden fruit.

4. Nonverbal Communication: Examine the significance of body language, facial expressions, and eye contact in conveying desire and building sexual tension. Provide tips for reading and responding to nonverbal cues, as well as techniques for using body language to communicate interest and attraction.

5. Verbal Seduction: Explore the art of verbal seduction, including the use of flirtatious banter, provocative language, and subtle innuendo to create tension and intrigue. Discuss the importance of tone, pacing, and timing in verbal exchanges, as well as strategies for building rapport and establishing a connection through conversation.

6. Creating Anticipation: Highlight the importance of building anticipation and delaying gratification to heighten desire. Discuss techniques for gradually escalating tension over time, such as teasing, anticipation-building activities, and the artful manipulation of desire through subtle cues and gestures.

By mastering these elements, one can cultivate a seductive allure that entices and captivates, drawing others into a world of tantalizing possibilities and irresistible desire.

Nurturing Desire and Passion

Nurturing desire and passion is a delicate art that requires patience, attentiveness, and a deep understanding of both oneself and one's partner. Here's a comprehensive exploration of the various aspects involved in fostering and sustaining the flames of desire and passion:

1. Understanding Desires: Begin by delving into the depths of your own desires and those of your partner. Take the time to explore what ignites passion within you, whether it's physical touch, emotional connection, or shared experiences. Likewise, encourage your partner to express their desires openly and honestly, creating a safe and supportive space for authentic communication.

2. Creating Intimacy: Cultivate intimacy in your relationship by prioritizing quality time together and fostering emotional connection. Share your thoughts, feelings, and vulnerabilities with one another, deepening your bond and strengthening your connection. Engage in activities that promote intimacy, such as cuddling, kissing, and engaging in meaningful conversations.

3. Sparking Excitement: Keep the spark alive in your relationship by introducing novelty and excitement into your routines. Plan surprise date nights, explore new hobbies together, or embark on spontaneous adventures. Embrace spontaneity and embrace new experiences, allowing yourselves to break free from the monotony of everyday life and reignite the flames of passion.

4. Physical Connection: Cultivate physical intimacy by prioritizing touch and affection in your

relationship. Hold hands, hug, kiss, and engage in sensual touch to deepen your physical connection and reignite passion. Explore each other's bodies with curiosity and reverence, discovering new erogenous zones and experimenting with different sensations.

5.Emotional Connection: Nurture emotional intimacy by being present and attentive to your partner's needs and desires. Show empathy, compassion, and understanding, and validate your partner's feelings and experiences. Create a supportive environment where both partners feel safe to express themselves authentically and openly.

6.Communication: Foster open and honest communication in your relationship, discussing your desires, fantasies, and boundaries openly and without judgment. Listen actively to your partner's needs and concerns, and be willing to compromise and find solutions that work for both of you. Practice active listening, empathy, and validation, and strive to understand your partner's perspective.

7. Self-Care: Prioritize self-care and self-love in your life, nurturing your own well-being and happiness. Take time to engage in activities that bring you joy and fulfillment, whether it's practicing mindfulness, pursuing hobbies, or spending time with loved ones. Cultivate a positive self-image and embrace your own unique beauty and worth,

allowing yourself to radiate confidence and self-assurance.

8.Adventurous Exploration: Embrace adventure and exploration in your relationship, both in and out of the bedroom. Try new things together, whether it's experimenting with different sexual positions or embarking on a spontaneous road trip. Embrace the unknown and embrace new experiences, allowing yourselves to grow and evolve together as a couple.

By nurturing desire and passion in your relationship, you can create a deep and lasting connection that enriches your lives and brings you closer together. By prioritizing intimacy, communication, and self-care, you can cultivate a relationship that is vibrant, fulfilling, and overflowing with love and passion.

Savoring The Thrill Of The Chase

Savoring the thrill of the chase is an invigorating experience that tantalizes the senses and stirs the soul. It's about fully embracing the excitement of pursuing what we desire and relishing in the anticipation of what's to come. Let's delve into how to immerse ourselves in the pursuit and relish every moment of the chase:

1. Embracing Anticipation: The journey commences with anticipation—an electric sensation that propels us forward with fervent enthusiasm. It's about eagerly anticipating the unknown and allowing ourselves to be swept away by the thrill of the chase. Anticipation heightens our senses, quickens our heartbeat, and fills us with a sense of eager expectation as we eagerly pursue our desires.

2. Cultivating Desire: At the heart of the chase lies desire—the primal force that propels us towards our goals. It's about tapping into our deepest yearnings and allowing them to ignite our passion and drive. Cultivating desire entails embracing our innermost longings and pursuing them with unyielding determination and passion.

3. Playing the Game: The chase is akin to a dance—a sophisticated game of strategy, finesse, and skill. It's about knowing when to advance and when to retreat, when to press forward and when to exercise patience. Playing the game involves navigating the intricacies of human interaction with confidence and grace, reveling in the exhilarating pursuit.

4. Savoring the Moment: Amidst the chase, it's crucial to pause and savor the experience—to fully immerse ourselves in the excitement of the pursuit

and cherish the journey as much as the destination. Savoring the moment requires presence, full engagement, and mindfulness of the sensations and emotions that accompany the chase.

5. Embracing Uncertainty: The thrill of the chase is inherently unpredictable—a rollercoaster ride of highs and lows, twists and turns. It's about embracing the ambiguity of the journey and surrendering to the exhilarating rush of adrenaline that accompanies it. Embracing uncertainty entails relinquishing control and allowing ourselves to be carried away by the excitement of the chase.

6. Celebrating Victory: Ultimately, the thrill of the chase culminates in triumph—the gratifying moment when our efforts are rewarded and our desires fulfilled. It's about celebrating our achievements and basking in the satisfaction of a job well done. Celebrating victory involves acknowledging our accomplishments with pride and gratitude, allowing ourselves to revel in the glow of success.

By savoring the thrill of the chase, we can fully immerse ourselves in the exhilaration of pursuing our desires and embrace the journey with open arms. It's about cherishing every moment, from the electrifying anticipation to the sweet taste of victory, and allowing ourselves to be fully present and engaged in the pursuit of our passions.

Chapter 6: Embodying the Femme Fatale: Unleashing Your Seductive Power

The Femme Fatale archetype has long captivated the imagination, embodying a potent blend of allure, mystery, and danger. To embrace this persona is to tap into the seductive power that lies within, captivating others with an irresistible charm and enigmatic allure. Here's a comprehensive guide to embodying the Femme Fatale:

1.Owning Your Sensuality: At the core of the Femme Fatale persona lies an unapologetic embrace of sensuality and sexuality. Embodying the Femme Fatale means owning your physicality with confidence, celebrating your curves, and reveling in the power of your allure. It's about recognizing that sensuality is a source of strength and empowerment, and allowing yourself to express it freely and unabashedly.

2.Cultivating Mystery: The Femme Fatale is shrouded in mystery, her enigmatic allure drawing others in like moths to a flame. Embrace the art of intrigue by cultivating an air of mystery around yourself. Keep others guessing with tantalizing hints and subtle suggestions, leaving them intrigued and captivated by the secrets you hold.

3. Mastering the Art of Seduction: Seduction is the Femme Fatale's greatest weapon, wielded with precision and finesse. Learn to entice and beguile with a glance, a touch, or a whispered word. Master the art of seductive communication, using body language, tone of voice, and suggestive language to create an irresistible allure that leaves others spellbound.

4. Embracing Independence: The Femme Fatale is a symbol of fierce independence, answering to no one but herself. Embrace your autonomy and self-reliance, refusing to be constrained by societal expectations or the opinions of others. Forge your own path with confidence and determination, embodying the spirit of a true Femme Fatale who answers to no one but herself.

5.Exuding Confidence: Confidence is the hallmark of the Femme Fatale, radiating from every pore and commanding attention wherever she goes. Cultivate an unwavering self-assurance that speaks volumes without uttering a word. Stand tall, walk with purpose, and exude an aura of confidence that draws others to you like a magnet.

6. Embracing Intelligence: The Femme Fatale is not just a seductress, but also a woman of intelligence and wit. Cultivate your intellect, engaging others in

stimulating conversation and showcasing your sharp wit and keen intellect. Embrace your intelligence as a source of power and sophistication, captivating others with your depth and insight.

7. Navigating Relationships: In matters of the heart, the Femme Fatale is a master strategist, navigating relationships with cunning and guile. Approach relationships with confidence and discernment, refusing to settle for anything less than what you deserve. Set boundaries, play by your own rules, and never compromise your independence or integrity for the sake of love.

8. Embracing Risk: The Femme Fatale is no stranger to risk, unafraid to flirt with danger in pursuit of her desires. Embrace the thrill of taking risks and stepping outside your comfort zone, knowing that true liberation lies on the other side of fear. Embody the spirit of adventure and embrace the unknown with courage and conviction.

By embodying the Femme Fatale, you unleash the full power of your seductive prowess, captivating others with your allure and leaving a trail of admirers in your wake. Embrace your sensuality, cultivate mystery, and wield the art of seduction with confidence and finesse, knowing that you hold the key to your own irresistible charm and magnetic allure.

Unleashing Your Inner Goddess: Embodying Divine Feminine Power

Your inner goddess is a beacon of strength, wisdom, and grace waiting to be unleashed. Embodying her essence is a journey of self-discovery and empowerment, allowing you to tap into the depths of your feminine energy. Here's how to embrace your inner goddess and harness her power:

1. Embrace Your Authenticity: Your inner goddess is uniquely you. Embrace every facet of your being—the light and the shadow, the strength and the vulnerability. Let go of societal expectations and embrace your authenticity with boldness and courage.

2. Connect with Nature: Nature is the embodiment of feminine energy—wild, untamed, and free. Spend time in nature, allowing its beauty to nourish your soul and reconnect you with your primal essence. Feel the earth beneath your feet, the wind in your hair, and the sun on your skin, and let nature remind you of your innate power.

3. Nurture Your Body: Your body is a temple, and your inner goddess resides within its sacred chambers. Honor your body with nourishing food, movement, and self-care rituals. Celebrate your

curves, your scars, and your imperfections as symbols of your unique beauty and strength.

4. Embrace Sensuality: Sensuality is the language of the goddess—a celebration of pleasure, passion, and desire. Indulge your senses with sensual experiences that awaken your divine feminine energy. Dance under the moonlight, luxuriate in a warm bath scented with essential oils, and savor the taste of decadent chocolate melting on your tongue.

5. Cultivate Inner Wisdom: Your inner goddess is a repository of ancient wisdom, whispering truths that resonate deep within your soul. Quiet your mind, listen to the whispers of your intuition, and trust in the wisdom that arises from within. Embrace your inner knowing and allow it to guide you on your journey with grace and clarity.

6. Celebrate Sisterhood: Sisterhood is the sacred bond that connects women across time and space. Celebrate the women in your life as embodiments of the divine feminine, honoring their strength, resilience, and beauty. Lift each other up, support each other's dreams, and hold space for each other's growth and transformation.

7. Express Creativity: Creativity is the essence of the goddess—an expression of divine inspiration and imagination. Allow your creativity to flow freely, expressing yourself through art, music, writing, or

any other creative outlet that speaks to your soul. Release self-doubt and judgment, and embrace the joy of creative expression as a sacred act of self-discovery and empowerment.

8. Radiate Love and Compassion: Love is the most potent force in the universe, and your inner goddess is a beacon of love and compassion. Radiate love outwardly, offering kindness, compassion, and empathy to yourself and others. Embrace the interconnectedness of all beings and cultivate a spirit of love that transcends boundaries and unites us all.

By embracing your inner goddess, you reclaim your divine feminine power and step into your true essence as a woman. Allow her light to shine brightly, illuminating your path with grace, wisdom, and love.

Embracing Your Sensuality and Sexuality: A Path to Self-Discovery and Empowerment

Embracing your sensuality and sexuality is a journey of self-discovery and empowerment—a celebration of the divine essence that resides within you. It's about honoring your body, embracing your desires, and reclaiming your power as a sensual, sexual being. Here's a comprehensive guide to embracing your sensuality and sexuality:

1. Honoring Your Body: Your body is a sacred vessel, the physical manifestation of your essence and spirit. Embrace your body with love and gratitude, honoring its curves, contours, and intricacies. Practice self-care rituals that nourish your body, such as massage, bathing, and skincare. Treat yourself with kindness and compassion, knowing that your body is a temple worthy of reverence and respect.

2. Exploring Your Desires: Your desires are an expression of your innermost needs and longings. Take the time to explore your desires without judgment or shame, allowing yourself to fully experience the pleasure and excitement they bring. Whether through self-pleasure, intimate connections, or erotic fantasies, give yourself

permission to indulge in what brings you joy and fulfillment.

3. Cultivating Sensuality: Sensuality is the language of the body—a celebration of pleasure, sensation, and intimacy. Cultivate your sensuality by engaging all of your senses, savoring the sights, sounds, smells, tastes, and textures that surround you. Allow yourself to be fully present in the moment, immersing yourself in the richness of sensory experience and delighting in the pleasures of the physical world.

4. Embracing Erotic Energy: Erotic energy is the life force that flows through you, fueling your creativity, vitality, and passion. Embrace your erotic energy as a source of power and vitality, allowing it to infuse every aspect of your life with passion and purpose. Cultivate practices that awaken your erotic energy, such as dance, breathwork, or tantra, and channel it into creative expression, personal growth, and intimate connection.

5.Navigating Intimate Relationships: Intimate relationships are an opportunity for growth, connection, and deepening intimacy. Navigate your relationships with honesty, authenticity, and open communication, expressing your desires and boundaries with clarity and confidence. Embrace vulnerability as a path to intimacy, allowing yourself to be seen, heard, and loved exactly as you are.

6. Healing Past Wounds: Past experiences and traumas can create barriers to embracing your sensuality and sexuality. Take the time to heal from past wounds, seeking support from therapists, coaches, or healers if needed. Practice self-compassion and forgiveness, releasing shame, guilt, and self-limiting beliefs that may be holding you back from fully embracing your sexuality.

7. Empowering Self-Expression: Your sexuality is a powerful form of self-expression, reflecting your unique desires, preferences, and identity. Empower yourself to express your sexuality authentically and unapologetically, without fear of judgment or criticism. Celebrate your sexual identity and orientation as a beautiful and integral part of who you are, and honor the diversity of human sexuality with compassion and acceptance.

8. Embracing Pleasure: Pleasure is your birthright—a natural and essential aspect of being human. Embrace pleasure as a guiding principle in your life, prioritizing activities, relationships, and experiences that bring you joy, satisfaction, and fulfillment. Allow yourself to revel in the simple pleasures of life, whether it's a delicious meal, a warm embrace, or a breathtaking sunset, and savor the richness of each moment with gratitude and appreciation.

By embracing your sensuality and sexuality, you reclaim your power as a sensual, sexual being, worthy of love, pleasure, and fulfillment. Embrace your desires, honor your body, and celebrate the divine essence that resides within you, knowing that your sexuality is a sacred gift to be cherished and embraced with reverence and joy.

Embracing Your Power Without Apology: A Journey to Self-Realization and Liberation

In a world that often seeks to diminish our power, embracing it without apology is an act of radical self-love and liberation. It's about stepping into our full potential, owning our strengths, and unapologetically asserting our worth. Here's a comprehensive guide to embracing your power without apology:

1. Recognizing Your Innate Worth: Your worth is not contingent upon external validation or approval. It's an intrinsic aspect of your being, rooted in your very existence. Recognize and honor your innate worthiness, acknowledging that you are deserving of love, respect, and dignity simply by virtue of being alive.

2. Owning Your Strengths: Each of us possesses unique strengths, talents, and abilities that contribute to the tapestry of humanity. Embrace and

celebrate your strengths without reservation, recognizing them as gifts to be shared with the world. Whether it's your creativity, resilience, intelligence, or compassion, own your strengths with pride and confidence.

3. Setting Boundaries: Boundaries are essential for protecting your energy, well-being, and autonomy. Set clear boundaries in your relationships and interactions, honoring your needs, values, and boundaries. Communicate your boundaries assertively and unapologetically, and enforce them with firmness and consistency.

4. Speaking Your Truth: Your truth is your most potent weapon in the journey to self-realization and empowerment. Speak your truth boldly and unapologetically, even when it feels uncomfortable or confrontational. Trust your voice, express your opinions, and assert your beliefs with clarity and conviction.

5. Embracing Self-Confidence: Self-confidence is the cornerstone of personal power. Cultivate self-confidence by affirming your worth, acknowledging your achievements, and embracing your inherent value. Stand tall, speak with conviction, and carry yourself with the assurance of someone who knows their worth.

6. Taking Ownership of Your Choices: You are the author of your own story, and every choice you

make shapes the narrative of your life. Take ownership of your choices without blame or regret, recognizing them as opportunities for growth and self-discovery. Trust yourself, follow your intuition, and embrace the power of agency.

7. Resisting External Validation: Your worth is not determined by the opinions or judgments of others. Resist the temptation to seek external validation or approval, and instead, cultivate self-validation from within. Trust your instincts, honor your intuition, and celebrate your accomplishments without seeking validation from others.

8. Embracing Imperfection: Perfection is an unattainable standard that only serves to undermine our sense of self-worth. Embrace your imperfections as beautiful and unique aspects of your humanity. Celebrate your flaws, vulnerabilities, and mistakes as opportunities for growth and self-compassion, and reject the pressure to conform to unrealistic ideals.

By embracing your power without apology, you reclaim your sovereignty, dignity, and agency as a human being. Stand unapologetically in your truth, honor your worth, and refuse to diminish yourself for the comfort or approval of others. Embrace your power with courage and conviction, knowing that you are worthy of love, respect, and success exactly as you are.

Conclusion: Embrace Your Journey

As we arrive at the culmination of this transformative odyssey, it's time to pause and reflect on the profound evolution that has unfolded. Embracing your power isn't merely a destination but a continuous voyage—a journey of self-discovery, empowerment, and profound self-acceptance.

Reflecting on the path traversed, take a moment to acknowledge the growth you've experienced. Remember the challenges surmounted, the obstacles overcome, and the triumphs celebrated. Each step forward, no matter how small, is a testament to your resilience, fortitude, and unwavering commitment to personal growth.

Amidst the reflection, celebrate your achievements, both monumental and minuscule. Whether it's asserting boundaries, vocalizing your truth, or embracing your sensuality, each milestone marks a pivotal moment in your journey toward self-realization. Take pride in your progress and the person you've become along the way.

Gratitude permeates the air, as you express appreciation for the myriad experiences, lessons, and individuals who have illuminated your path. From supportive friends and family to inspirational mentors and teachers, their presence has been a guiding light, igniting your inner flame and propelling you forward.

In the present moment, immerse yourself fully—embracing the now as the culmination of your journey. Release the shackles of the past and relinquish the anxieties of the future, as you bask in the beauty of the present. Life's impermanence becomes a poignant reminder to savor each moment, cherishing it as a precious gift.

With a steadfast commitment to growth, pledge to continue your journey with an insatiable curiosity and unwavering determination. Embrace the unknown with open arms, recognizing it as an opportunity for growth, expansion, and boundless possibility. Trust in the wisdom of the universe to guide you, knowing that the journey of self-discovery is a lifelong adventure filled with infinite potential.

As you navigate the vast expanse of your inner landscape, remember to share your light with the world. Your journey isn't just for you—it's a beacon of hope and inspiration for others embarking on their own path of self-discovery. Shine brightly, radiate kindness, and be a force of positive change in the world.

In the fabric of life, every journey is unique, every path distinct. Embrace your journey with an open heart, a courageous spirit, and an unwavering belief in your inherent worthiness. For in embracing your journey, you embrace your power—and in embracing your power, you embrace the infinite possibilities that lie within.

Appendix: Practical Exercises and Resources

In this appendix, you'll find a treasure trove of practical exercises and valuable resources designed to deepen your journey of self-discovery, empowerment, and seduction mastery. These exercises are crafted to enhance your understanding, cultivate your skills, and ignite your passion as you embrace your feminine power and navigate the intricacies of seduction.

Practical Exercises:

1. Mirror Work: Spend time in front of a mirror, gazing into your own eyes with love and acceptance. Affirm your worth, beauty, and strength aloud, reinforcing positive self-talk and building self-confidence.

2. Journaling Prompts: Set aside time for reflective journaling, using prompts to explore your desires, fears, and aspirations. Dive deep into your innermost thoughts and feelings, allowing your pen to guide you on a journey of self-discovery.

3. Sensory Exploration: Engage your senses in sensory exploration exercises designed to heighten your awareness and enhance your sensual experience. Experiment with different scents, textures, tastes, and sounds, reveling in the rich tapestry of sensory delights that surround you.

4. Body Language Practice: Practice embodying confident body language through exercises such as power posing, assertive posture, and graceful movement. Become attuned to the subtle signals your body sends and learn to express confidence and allure through your physical presence.

5.Communication Skills: Hone your communication skills through role-playing exercises, active listening practice, and assertiveness training. Learn to express your desires, set boundaries, and engage in meaningful conversations with authenticity and clarity.

Resources:

1. Books: Explore a curated selection of books on feminine empowerment, seduction psychology, and personal development. Dive into timeless classics and contemporary gems that offer valuable insights and practical guidance on your journey.

2. Online Courses: Enroll in online courses and workshops led by experts in the fields of seduction,

communication, and personal growth. Access video tutorials, interactive exercises, and downloadable resources to deepen your learning and expand your skills.

3. Community Support: Connect with like-minded individuals in online forums, support groups, and social media communities dedicated to feminine empowerment and seduction mastery. Share experiences, seek advice, and find inspiration in the collective wisdom of your peers.

4. Coaching and Mentorship: Consider seeking guidance from experienced coaches or mentors who specialize in feminine empowerment, seduction, and personal transformation. Receive personalized support, accountability, and guidance as you navigate your journey of self-discovery and growth.

5. Podcasts and Audio Resources: Tune into podcasts and audio resources featuring interviews, discussions, and guided meditations on topics related to feminine empowerment, seduction, and personal development. Immerse yourself in inspiring content that uplifts and empowers you on your journey.

With these practical exercises and valuable resources at your disposal, you'll have everything you need to deepen your understanding, cultivate your skills, and unleash your full feminine power.

Embrace these opportunities for growth and transformation, knowing that each step you take brings you closer to embodying the confident, captivating woman you were always meant to be.